3 POWERFUL TIPS TO OPTIMUM KIDNEY FUNCTIONS.

Discovery the essentials to kidney performance.

Dr DOUGLAS JASON

Copyright © (DR DOUGLAS JASON) 2022. All rights reserved

3 POWERFUL TIPS TO OPTIMUM KIDNEY FUNCTIONS

Before this document is duplicated or reproduced in any manner, the publisher's consent must be gained.

Therefore, the contents within can neither be stored electronically, transferred, nor kept in a database. Neither in part nor in full can the document be copied, scanned, faxed,

3 POWERFUL TIPS TO OPTIMUM KIDNEY FUNCTIONS

or retained without approval from the publisher or creator.

3 POWERFUL TIPS TO OPTIMUM KIDNEY FUNCTIONS

TABLE OF CONTENT

ABOUT THE AUTHOR

INTRODUCTION

3 POWERFUL TIPS TO OPTIMUM KIDNEY FUNCTIONS

TABLE OF CONTENT

3 POWERFUL TIPS TO OPTIMUM KIDNEY FUNCTIONS

Discovery the essentials to kidney performance.

3 POWERFUL TIPS TO OPTIMUM KIDNEY FUNCTIONS

INTRODUCTION

CHAPTER 1
Keep yourself hydrated.

CHAPTER 2
Remain active

CHAPTER 3

3 POWERFUL TIPS TO OPTIMUM KIDNEY FUNCTIONS

Give up smoking

CONCLUSION

3 POWERFUL TIPS TO OPTIMUM KIDNEY FUNCTIONS

ABOUT THE AUTHOR

Dr. Douglas Jason is a certified dietician who has a strong passion for wellness and a big eagerness to help people all over the world. He uses healthy food, herbs, spices, and other useful tools to help mankind realize its overall goal of optimum health

3 POWERFUL TIPS TO OPTIMUM KIDNEY FUNCTIONS

INTRODUCTION

The kidneys are essential organs that carry out several key bodily processes.

3 POWERFUL TIPS TO OPTIMUM KIDNEY FUNCTIONS

The kidneys are essential organs that carry out many crucial bodily activities.
The kidneys are essential organs that carry out several crucial bodily activities. In the US, about one-third of adults are at risk of having the renal disease. Kidney disease is

3 POWERFUL TIPS TO OPTIMUM KIDNEY FUNCTIONS

more common in those who take long-term drugs or have disorders like diabetes or hypertension. Unfortunately, the majority of kidney disease sufferers take a very long time to discover any symptoms. As a result, individuals would already have suffered a great

3 POWERFUL TIPS TO OPTIMUM KIDNEY FUNCTIONS

deal of irreparable harm by the time they receive a diagnosis, leaving them with only two options: dialysis or a kidney transplant.

The kidneys carry out some tasks, including:

maintain a healthy balance of salt and water in the body

3 POWERFUL TIPS TO OPTIMUM KIDNEY FUNCTIONS

Remove different toxins and pollutants from the body
Maintain a healthy balance of electrolytes in the body, including sodium, potassium, magnesium, and phosphorus.
maintain ideal blood pressure
Ensure strong bones by utilizing vitamin D

3 POWERFUL TIPS TO OPTIMUM KIDNEY FUNCTIONS

Keep the body's red blood cell count at a healthy level. Kidney illnesses can be caused by some factors. These consist of:

elevated blood pressure
Diabetes

3 POWERFUL TIPS TO OPTIMUM KIDNEY FUNCTIONS

smoking cigarettes

Obesity

Heart conditions

renal disease running in families

using some medications for an extended period, such as nonsteroidal anti-inflammatory drugs (NSAIDs) (painkillers)

3 POWERFUL TIPS TO OPTIMUM KIDNEY FUNCTIONS

Multiple myeloma and lupus are examples of autoimmune disorders

renal stones

recurring infections of the urinary tract

older age

Particularly if you are at risk for renal problems, it is crucial to

3 POWERFUL TIPS TO OPTIMUM KIDNEY FUNCTIONS

take care of your kidneys and get frequent checkups.

3 POWERFUL TIPS TO OPTIMUM KIDNEY FUNCTIONS

CHAPTER 1

Keep yourself hydrated.

Maintaining the health of your kidneys requires drinking

3 POWERFUL TIPS TO OPTIMUM KIDNEY FUNCTIONS

plenty of fluids. The ideal fluid intake is influenced by some variables, including physical activity, weather, and medical conditions. If you are healthy and living in a comfortable climate, it is recommended that you drink about two liters of fluids every day. To find out

3 POWERFUL TIPS TO OPTIMUM KIDNEY FUNCTIONS

what level of fluid you require, speak with your doctor.

3 POWERFUL TIPS TO OPTIMUM KIDNEY FUNCTIONS

CHAPTER 2

Remain active

Risk factors for kidney disease, such as obesity,

3 POWERFUL TIPS TO OPTIMUM KIDNEY FUNCTIONS

hypertension, and diabetes, are reduced by regular physical activity.
Maintain a healthy weight since renal illnesses may be more likely to develop if you are overweight or obese.
EAT HEALTHY: Fruits and vegetables, as well as

3 POWERFUL TIPS TO OPTIMUM KIDNEY FUNCTIONS

avoiding processed and greasy foods, will help you maintain the health of your kidneys. Keep your daily salt intake to 5–6 g maximum. How to control your blood pressure: Check your blood pressure frequently. In agreement with your doctor,

3 POWERFUL TIPS TO OPTIMUM KIDNEY FUNCTIONS

take the proper drugs and start living a healthy lifestyle. Control your blood sugar levels: Many persons with diabetes receive a late diagnosis. Based on any potential risk factors for diabetes, you should routinely check your blood sugar.

3 POWERFUL TIPS TO OPTIMUM KIDNEY FUNCTIONS

Controlling blood sugar levels can help avoid diabetes-related kidney damage.

3 POWERFUL TIPS TO OPTIMUM KIDNEY FUNCTIONS

3 POWERFUL TIPS TO OPTIMUM KIDNEY FUNCTIONS

CHAPTER 3

Give up smoking

The kidneys are harmed by smoking in any capacity, including vaping and passive smoking. Additionally, smoking

3 POWERFUL TIPS TO OPTIMUM KIDNEY FUNCTIONS

can raise your chances of kidney cancer and heart problems.

Avoid taking over-the-counter painkillers frequently: NSAIDs and other painkillers used over an extended period can harm your kidneys.

3 POWERFUL TIPS TO OPTIMUM KIDNEY FUNCTIONS

Check the health of your kidneys if you are in danger. To rule out the emergence of renal illnesses, those with risk factors such as diabetes, high blood pressure, obesity, and a family history of kidney disease must undergo routine physical examinations. If you

3 POWERFUL TIPS TO OPTIMUM KIDNEY FUNCTIONS

have diabetes or high blood pressure, getting tested for urine protein or microalbuminuria (trace protein in the urine) every six months is an excellent approach to tracking your kidney function. A positive test

3 POWERFUL TIPS TO OPTIMUM KIDNEY FUNCTIONS

results in kidney damage, which is still treatable.

3 POWERFUL TIPS TO OPTIMUM KIDNEY FUNCTIONS

CONCLUSION

From person to person, the chance of acquiring renal illnesses can change. Certain

3 POWERFUL TIPS TO OPTIMUM KIDNEY FUNCTIONS

unchangeable variables could put you at risk, including age, genetics, and family history of kidney disease. You can reduce your chance of acquiring kidney illnesses by controlling controllable factors including a healthy diet and lifestyle.

3 POWERFUL TIPS TO OPTIMUM KIDNEY FUNCTIONS

www.ingramcontent.com/pod-product-compliance
Lightning Source LLC
Chambersburg PA
CBHW050325220526
45465CB00005B/2129